The Science of Sleep

Learn How To Naturally Fall Asleep Faster, Stay Asleep Longer, Improve Sleep Disorders and Revitalize Your Life.

Table of Contents

thought of as universal. As befitting its nature, it is presented without assurance regarding its prolonged validity or interim quality. Trademarks that are mentioned are done without written consent and can in no way be considered an endorsement from the trademark holder.

Introduction

Congratulations on downloading *The Science of Sleep* and thank you for doing so.

The following chapters will discuss many elements of sleep. We'll cover topics such as what sleep is, and what scientists do and don't know about it. Sleep is an incredibly important physiological function, as necessary for life as food and water.

Sleep comes and goes in phases, cycles. "Biological Clock" and "Circadian Rhythms" are a few things you'll learn about.

You'll also find much useful information about how much sleep you need, why you need it, and ways to get more if you feel like you aren't getting enough.

Sleep is so simple, and yet it can be so complicated. It's often the first thing we sacrifice when we find ourselves without enough hours in the day. How many times have you heard the old saying, "there just aren't enough hours in the day?" It is so true! And yet, within the hours that we do have, getting plenty of sleep should be at the top of the priority list. As you read on, you'll discover precisely why, and more.

There are plenty of books on this subject on the market, thanks again for choosing this one! Every effort was made to ensure it is full of as much useful information as possible, please enjoy

Chapter One: Theories Behind the Science of Sleep

"To sleep, perchance to dream" from Hamlet by William Shakespeare For everything we know about sleep, there is so much that we do not understand.

For much of the history of mankind, little has been understood about sleep. It wasn't until the 1900's that scientist began to make discoveries about its complex nature. In 1911 the first book dealing with the science of sleep was published. Written by French Scientist Henry Pieron, "Le probleme physiologique du sommeil," the English translation for this title is "the physiological problem of sleep," and the book is credited as the first text to link sleep to physiology. Pieron is widely given credit for the integration of a modern approach to the study of sleep. Another key player in the field was a man referred to in sleep studies circles as "the father of American sleep research," Dr. Nathaniel Kleitman. He was among the first to perform sleep studies on different populations. In 1953 he and a colleague and student, Dr. Eugene Aserinsky, discovered what is known as REM or "rapid eye movement," which is actually a phase within the sleep cycle. You will read more about sleep cycles later.

Another of Kleitmans students, Dr. William C. Dement, in his own research, was able to establish the connection between REM sleep and dreaming. Dr. Dement also published a paper on the cyclic organization of sleep in cats. According to sleep research history, this particular finding, that sleep cycles exist in species other than humans, is credited for having inspired vast amounts of research in the field over the next twenty years. This research eventually led to the discovery by a man named Michel Jouvet that REM (rapid eye movement) sleep is actually an independent state of alertness for which he coined the phrase "Paradoxical Sleep." More will be revealed about REM sleep later when the topic of the different phases of sleep is discussed.

Sleep apnea, a potentially dangerous sleep disorder characterized by the stopping and starting of breathing during sleep, loud snoring, and feeling exhausted despite having slept the full night was discovered during a sleep study in Europe in 1965 by a man named H. Gastaut and the colleagues he was working with at the time. This led to further controlled studies on the relationship between sleep and the body's main functions. Sleep Apnea will also be covered in more detail.

The field of sleep study has broadened and continued since these major breakthroughs. Today there is a vast field of sleep research with subgroups studying almost every area imaginable. There are many published works dedicated to the science of sleep.

There are countless areas to be studied and researched regarding sleep, perhaps with some of the most basic going hand in hand with what could be considered among the most important. To name a few:

- What exactly is sleep?

- What happens when we sleep, physiologically?

- What happens to us when we are deprived of sleep?

- Are there any negative consequences for those who sleep "too much?" How is "too much," or for that matter, too little, defined?

- Can sleep deprivation have benefits?

- Can long-term sleep deprivation be harmful to one's help?

- What are the differences between those who sleep well and those who do not?

I have just barely touched on the beginnings of the elements scientists desire to understand about sleep. The complete list alone could likely comprise an entire chapter.

I'd like to begin here by presenting the question: why do we need sleep in the first place?

It is estimated that most humans spend nearly a third of their life sleeping, and while there may not be an exact definitive answer for a reason, scientific theories abound. Much like the fundamental actions of eating, drinking, and breathing, sleep does serve a critical role in our health and well-being. Getting optimal sleep (the right kind at the right times and enough of it) is far more important than most people realize.

Sleeping is regulated by an internal drive, just as hunger is. Just as going without food makes us feel hungry, then going without sleep makes us feel tired.

Although scientists have many credible theories explaining why we sleep, there is no set in stone evidence of the absolute correctness of any of them. What's considered to be true is that there is more than one correct theory. Here we'll take a look at some theories:

Inactivity Theory

One of the earliest of the theories, this one is based on simple evolution. It suggests that humans sleep for much the same reason animals slept in the wild. Inactivity at night served as a function to keep the animal out of harms' way in the darkness. Shutting down and remaining still at night prevented these creatures from either having accidents in the dark or becoming prey to other animals. This theory posits that this process of shutting down began as a behavioral strategy and then, through evolution, became sleep.

Energy Conservation Theory

This theory also pertains to evolution, our ancestors, animals and the process known as natural selection. As it turns out one of the most powerful components in natural selection is being able to utilize our energy resources to their maximum benefit. According to the Energy Conservation Theory, the primary function of sleep is to reduce energy expenditure during the times when it would make the least sense to search for food. Our metabolism needs when we are asleep are much less than when we are awake. While sleeping, we don't burn nearly as many calories as we do awake, and additionally, when we are asleep, our bodies maintain lower temperatures, thus conserving energy.

Restorative or Rejuvenate Theory

This theory is the one I would have written a version of had I been asked to write on this subject without any research. In other words, it's the most common-sense theory to me. Not that the other theories don't make sense or apply. That's irrelevant because it's already been established that there is no one agreed-upon universal theory for why we sleep and that it's more likely a combination of several or even many. This one makes simple sense. When I've had a long busy day and night comes, I begin to feel tired, if I wasn't already tired even earlier in the day. If I push through that tiredness, perhaps I'm writing a piece and working against a deadline…I can feel, as I become more tired, many physiological changes taking place. My cognitive skills decline. I develop "brain-fog." I have less physical energy. Sometimes getting up to get a last drink of water before I retire feels like much more of an energy expenditure than it should be. Eventually, at times, I can feel myself literally struggling to keep my eyes open.

After I sleep, and I'm not always able to, I wake in a totally different place mentally, physically and even emotionally. Yes, I don't think I'm the only one who has noticed, sleep deprivation tends to make one feel more emotional. It does this, especially with children. If you're a parent, you'll know straight away what I'm referring to. Ever used or heard of the term "Crazy Hour?" My brother and sister-in-law use that term to describe the insanity that is the hour before their children's bedtime. The more tired children get, the more they are prone to act out. Adults experience something of a similar nature.

While we may not be running around jumping on the furniture in our pajamas or throwing a screaming fit because one of our siblings "hit us," we may certainly tend to become grumpy or feel lackluster, at the least and for many, it can be much worse than that. Sleep is not just an important physiological function. In a sense, it's a panacea for most of what ails us. What do most people have a tendency to do when they're ill? Well...sleep, yes, sleep. Why? Because it's restorative, it helps brings up back up to par, so to speak. We go to sleep exhausted and defeated and wake up to a new day, energized and restored.

A full restful night of sleep can feel like a tall glass of ice water after a hard run on a hot summer day. Restorative and invigorating. A good night of sleep is like a reset back to a healthy baseline.

This theory is not simply mine based on my own subjective and objective experiences, it's been researched and verified within studies both on humans and animals. In studies, animals that were deprived entirely of sleep lost all immune functions and died within a matter of weeks. Other conclusive findings have supported the fact that many essential functions in the body such as muscle growth, tissue repair, protein synthesis and the release of growth hormones occur primarily and sometimes only while we are sleeping.

Athletes have long known that while the demanding work is done out on the track, or on the field or the rink or in the ring, that the processes that build muscle and generate new levels of fitness cannot happen without sleep. Sleep is a key component of growth and muscle regeneration and building.

During our waking hours, neurons in our brains produce adenosine which leads to the perception of being tired. As we sleep, our bodies clear this adenosine from our systems, giving us the chance to feel rested when we wake.

Brain Plasticity Theory

Could sleep be powerful enough to actually change our brains? Recent and conclusive research sets forth that this is true. The Brain Plasticity Theory, while yet not entirely understood, posits just such a theory. It has been proven that sleep plays a key role in the developments of the brains of infants and young children. If you pause for a moment and consider this, that would explain why infants sleep more than perhaps any other humans of more advanced ages. Their brains have the most developing to do, in a relatively brief period of time if you consider an average life-span. A connection in adults has also been established, between the number of hours of sleep amassed and the plasticity of their brains. This is most evident during tests involving total hours of sleep and considering the brain's ability to absorb new information accordingly.

As I alluded to previously, none of these theories directly

and completely answer the question, "why do humans need sleep?" and yet much legitimate study has been conducted, and these theories do go far towards putting forth a so-called "educated guess" for a question science may never have a precise answer to.

What is obvious and unarguable to most is how much better we all feel when we are getting an adequate amount of sleep. Even people who sleep well, I'm sure, have found themselves experiencing a night of bad sleep here or there. The difference in how we feel the day after a "bad" night of sleep, or rather a night where we didn't get enough, although subjective for each of us, tends to carry plenty of common denominators.

Have you ever had an important test to take or a presentation to give the next day and tossed and turned and were not able to sleep the night before? From the moment we wake up after not getting too much sleep, things just simply seem off. For some people their appetite is affected, they might not be hungry for breakfast as normal and yet later as the day wears on they may find themselves craving starchy, carb- and sugar-laden food. Unhealthy food. This is the body's way of trying to compensate for the lack of energy. Some people can drink a little extra caffeine and be fine, but others will simply feel tired and jittery from too much caffeine. Lack of sleep can cause brain fog, memory lapses. It can cause a person to become irritable or short with people when it's not normally in their nature to be that way. Sometimes not getting enough sleep can even cause a person to feel depressed.

Obviously, if you have a serious sleep disorder, which we will be addressing later than you may need to take some measures above and beyond what the average person might have to do.

If your lack of sleep is a temporary situation, brought on by something acute, sometimes a simple catnap will help. A catnap is a term used to describe a very short nap. There have been plenty of studies that have shown that when a person is tired, a twenty-minute nap can actually be more beneficial than a longer one. There is some solid science behind why a "power nap" or a "cat nap" can be so helpful.

A power nap, or catnap as some like to call it, is a short nap you take during the day (ideally between 1:00 to 4:00 PM) which should last anywhere from ten to thirty minutes. Any longer and you run the risk of developing "sleep inertia" — that unpleasant groggy feeling that takes a considerable amount of time to shake off. And naps later than 4:00 PM can disrupt your regular nighttime sleep. But a power nap can go a long way towards making you feel refreshed and helping you get through the rest of the day.

If you are not a person with a sleep disorder and yet you sometimes get behind on your sleep, chances are you're not going to suffer too many negative effects unless it turns into a chronic issue. There are two things that studies have shown conflicting results about. One is this the theory about whether or not sleep is a "bankable" commodity. In other words, can sleeping extra time for a few nights before a night when you know you're going to be sleep deprived help? I say a little extra sleep never hurt either way, so go for it. Another area of sleep research where there have been some different results come out of studies is on whether or not you can "catch up" on lost sleep. The general hypothesis is that it doesn't work that way.

This hypothesis happens to be one I can speak to from personal experience as a lifelong insomniac. My insomnia has shown itself in many ways through the years. I've had extended periods where, with the help of a supplement or even prescription medication, I could get four or five hours of sleep and yet always seemed to wake at three a.m. no matter what. I've also experienced entire sleepless nights, and many nights where I was only able to sleep two or three hours. I've gone through phases where I could catch a daytime nap, and there have been times when it was impossible to fall asleep during the day. My battle with sleeplessness has been strange, but I certainly don't believe I'm the only one who has experienced it in this manner.

On the subject of whether or not it's possible to catch up on lost sleep, my vote would be: yes, sort of. I had had times when, after three or four particularly bad nights, for whatever reason, perhaps simple exhaustion, I was able to get an entire night of "good" sleep. I'm here to tell you the restorative power of that one night, for me, sure gave me a subjective feeling that is somewhat possible to "catch-up" on lost sleep.

I've never been able to test the theory about banking sleep. If I could do that I probably would not be the insomniac that I am.

Chapter Two: How Much Sleep Do We Need, Anyway?

"Sleep is the golden chain that binds health and our bodies together." - Thomas Dekker

How much sleep is enough? There is no salient answer to that question. It's different across the board for everyone. Some people can survive and thrive on three hours of sleep per night. Others might struggle if they get less than eight or nine. There are, however, target numbers of hours of nightly sleep to aim for of people in different age groups.

It's not always easy. In this crazy busy world that we exist it in, sleep is often treated like a luxury instead of the extremely important necessity that it is.

It's true that a strong correlation has been made between the age of a person and determining the number of hours of sleep per night to be considered ideal. Many newborn babies sleep as much as sixteen or seventeen hours out of every twenty-four, waking primarily only to eat and bond with their parents. Since babies spend most of the time in the womb asleep, newborns sleep so much as part of a natural transitioning process into their new world, and also because they are growing and developing at an astonishingly faster rate than they ever will again.

Babies and Sleep

Most babies do not settle into a regular sleep cycle until at least six months of age, some longer than that, and there are even those rare newborns who seem to sleep through the night as early as their first few nights home from the hospital. It is more likely though, for a newborn to awaken every few hours to eat, as their tiny stomachs cannot hold enough nutrition to fill their needs for much longer. During their first few months, babies experience the greatest of life's transitions, that of entering the world after spending nine months inside the womb of their mother. This is no minor change. Inside a mother's womb is a warm and comfortable and peaceful place to be. It's difficult to imagine another set of circumstances more conducive to sleep.

As babies emerge into this life and grow and change daily, at first, they sleep almost constantly both as a way to hold on to the comfort and memory of their mother's wombs but perhaps most importantly, to begin their growth process. The two most crucial factors in a newborns life are food and sleep.
Parents should not be concerned about a newborn baby's sleep habits unless they seem problematic, in which case they should be discussed with the baby's pediatrician.

Otherwise, simply let the process flow. It's normal for some babies to sleep as much as eighteen hours per day. Enjoy the extra time your newborn sleeps to catch up on much-needed rest for yourself.

It's not uncommon for babies to be born with their days and night reversed. Some babies will want to spend their "awake" time at night. This can make it hard for parents who already tend to be sleep deprived. If this happens, try to

make sure that your home is filled with light during the day.
Also, in the daytime when baby wakes to eat, try to make
that a stimulatory experience. Talk to them in a cheery voice,
be very alert with them. Playing music in the background is
a clever idea. Oppositely, at night, make feeding time's dark
and quiet, with no ambient noise. It usually doesn't take
babies long to find their personal circadian rhythms even if
they tend to be born backward. As a parent, simply try not to
be frustrated and get the sleep you can whenever you can.

It can take up to six months for a baby to establish their own
personal circadian rhythm. The most key factor is that your
baby is gaining weight and appears healthy. Of course,
regular check-ups and consultations with your baby's
Pediatrician will be at play during this time as well. If your
baby's doctor declares him or her healthy, and your baby
seems objectively healthy at home, try not to worry,
regardless of the sleep patterns he or she is exhibiting. As
previously mentioned, rest up as much as you can yourself.
You're going to need it.

Children

According to a sleep study following eleven-thousand
children, correlations were shown between improper
amounts of sleep in the first three years of their lives and
negatively impacted skills pertaining to reading, spatial
awareness, and math. The children were followed over time,
and these results proved to be significant through ages seven
and beyond. Another particularly interesting component that
emerged from the same study was that girls were more

impacted than boys. A study published in 2008 in the Canadian journal *Sleep* concluded that infants who regularly slept less than ten hours a night prior to age three were more at risk for developing ADHD and more likely to manifest problems pertaining to basic language and reading skills.

Babies, children's and teens, in general, require more sleep than adults, especially older adults. They are developing physically and mentally at lightning speed, and sleep is perhaps the most vital component of this development. Additionally, they are learning at a high rate, and spend their time constantly influenced by external stimuli. Sleep is the only restorative counter to all that activity. Parents don't have a set way to know how much sleep a child requires, so trial, error, and guesswork must come in to play. It is true, however, that so much as an hour or two of missed sleep here or there can make an impact on a child's development. Not only can their development be impacted but their behavior (and the peace of mind of parents everywhere.)

As adults, when we tire we relax, wind down. It becomes harder to stay alert and focus. We long for the comfort of our pajamas and our beds and to put the day behind us.

Paradoxically though, the more tired a child becomes, often the more "wound up" they will get. Overtired children tend to nonsensically resist bedtime. As most of you have been parents know, this phenomenon can turn in to a serious battle, one that causes much grief.

Researchers have found that health conditions can deprive children of sleep. Even conditions such as sleep apnea, once very much thought to exist in adults only, can actually present in children as well. Studies have been so conclusive in this area that the American Academy of Pediatrics recommends that all children be screened for this condition during regular wellness check-ups. Most especially those children who appear to be exhibiting abnormalities in their sleep patterns.

Children, when sleeping, spend the majority of time in a slow wave, or "deep" sleep. Studies link this type of sleep to brain development. It has been proven that REM (rapid eye movement) sleep contributes greatly to development in specific areas of the brain related to how we visualize the world around us.

Infants who are no longer newborns should still sleep from twelve to fourteen hours per day. This is most imperative because their bodies and brains are actually still forming. A child between three and six should be getting ten to twelve hours, and children between the ages of seven to twelve should still be getting close to ten hours of sleep per night.

Children: Kids aged twelve through eighteen should be getting eight or nine hours of sleep. Often kids between these ages are in a constant state of sleep deprivation since activities with friends and demands from school, and other commitments take away from the hours in the day that are available for sleep.

The need for children to get the proper amount of sleep cannot be stressed enough. Not only are all kinds of things going on internally from a developmental standpoint, but children need to be alert so that they can be in the best position to learn at school.

Children operating on a sleep deficit will not be able to concentrate or absorb and store information as those who are running on a full tank, or fully rested, in other words. Lack of sleep can also make life at school more difficult for children from a behavioral and disciplinary standpoint. Lack of sleep in children causes them to be much quicker to respond inappropriately to normal situations that take place throughout the day. Bad temper, crankiness, and disobedience can all be direct results of sleep deprivation in children. For that matter, the same can be said for adults.

It is important to understand that for anyone, children or adult, sleep deprivation is cumulative and ongoing lack of sleep can cause chronic negative results.

The most recent national poll shows that more than eighty-seven percent of American high school students get far less than the recommended eight to ten hours of sleep per night. In a detailed report in 2014, the American Academy of Pediatrics called the problem of tired teens a "public health epidemic."

That lack of sleep in teens is not only a threat to their success as students but to their health and safety as well. Lack of ability to concentrate is a major concern in sleep deprivation. The number of children of high school age who drive cars is higher than ever before. Drowsy driving is a serious risk. Children who suffer from sleep depression are at higher risk of depression, anxiety, and even suicidal thoughts. The pressure brought on from being a high school student is already so incredibly demanding. Factor in chronic sleep deprivation and there are going to be problems.

Teenagers have a natural tendency to go to sleep later. It's not uncommon for the demands of their homework alone to keep them up until midnight. Homework aside, modern technology, computers and computer games, social media, instant messenger and chat rooms have introduced a way for teens to be "social" far longer than they should every night of the week without leaving the comfort of their homes. Many teenagers, because they are much more interested in instant gratification and don't yet have a fully formed concept of delayed gratification, will sacrifice the hours of sleep easily to enjoy the evening socializing with their friends. Then, of course, there is still the homework.

Chronically falling asleep too late, then being forced to arise too early does not allow for enough of the deep sleep and productive rapid eye movement sleep we need so badly to restore us on every level. As teenagers spend their weeks this way, each night that they miss out on badly needed sleep can make the next worse than the last until the accumulated effects of missed sleep put them into a "sleep-debt" they can't work their way out of. Especially since after a week at school comes the weekend, and while some high school children sleep in late on Saturday and Sunday mornings, it doesn't always do enough to make up for the tendency of having stayed up much later the nights before.

High school children are still busy on the weekend with extracurricular activities, time spent with friends and family obligations.

Teens and sleep is a problem that may never be solved. The demands on them and their lifestyles simply aren't conducive to see them be able to get enough sleep. It would be nice to live in a reality where the plight of teenagers and sleep could be taken more seriously. It's hard to know what could fix the problem. Four-day school weeks? School days that start later, perhaps even ending later. A longer day at school might be better if it meant less or no homework.

This is an area where parents really need to step up to the plate and take on their own share of responsibility in the situation. The electronics kids are allowed to have from such young ages do not help the problem with sleep. Tired parents sending their children to bed when, in the bedrooms of the children there exist televisions, video game players, computers and phones that most teenagers have, does not help the situation.

As the parent who steps in and tries very hard to rearrange the factors in a teens life that are contributing to chronic sleep debt, and therefore putting their health at risk and even their safety in danger, you won't win any popularity contests. In this world we live in, that would not be an easy chore. However, your children are worth it, and you are, in fact, the parent and the "boss," theoretically at least, while your child is a minor living in your home.

Adults: The amount of sleep adults need to function in a healthy manner seems to vary widely. The general consensus seems to be seven to nine hours, or seven to eight hours for "older," adults, aged sixty-four and older.

This guideline seems like a reasonable one. I know many adults who function fine on eight hours of sleep. The problem is, I don't know many who get that much. Many people average more like four to six hours per night.

Sleep can be tricky. Some people can sleep well under the recommended amount and still feel and function fine, and yet, are those people putting themselves at risk for all of the things that can happen when a sleep deficit is built up over year after year?

Since we undergo so many critical processes for the health of our brains and bodies while we sleep, shouldn't we be trying to get more even if we can "get by" on less?

Through extensive studies scientists have actually pinpointed higher risk percentages for certain diseases directly correlated to lack of sleep:

Alzheimer's: In a 2013 study conducted at John's Hopkins University researchers found that poor sleep habits can be a cause of Alzheimer's Disease. Furthermore, this same study concluded that lack of sleep can expedite progression of the disease.

The study was initiated by previous research, which posited that sleep was essential to the elimination of waste-like buildup that accumulated in the brain called "cerebral waste."

Other studies have strongly indicated that as we sleep our brain eliminates unneeded and unwanted components. If we don't sleep enough, what happens to those components that do not get eliminated. What happens to a brain full of "cerebral waste," when there is no way for it to get dumped?

Prostate Cancer: In men between the ages of sixty-seven and ninety-six, sixty percent more of them with sleep problems developed Prostate Cancer than within those who did not exhibit any trouble with sleep. Additionally, it was found that in the same group the cancer was likely to progress to a more advanced stage.

Other cancers have also been identified to be more likely to develop in both men and women who don't sleep enough.

The conclusions are mostly based on the role that melatonin plays in the suppression of growth in tumors. Since melatonin is produced at the highest level while we sleep, chronically deprived people would not be able to manufacture enough of this hormone naturally.

Heart Disease: This condition has long been widely known to have a direct link to sleep. Many extensive studies have been conducted over the years. In a study that took place in Russia, of six-hundred and fifty-seven Russian men over a span of fourteen years it was found that two-thirds of those who eventually experienced a heart attack also had a sleep disorder. In the same study, the men with sleep disorders experienced strokes at a rate of four times higher than the men who didn't have trouble with their sleep.

These are incredibly significant findings and should be reason enough alone to inspire anyone to try harder to get the recommended amount of sleep, or to get help for their problems with sleep.

Obesity and Diabetes rates are also higher in those with sleep disorders. Additionally, and not surprisingly, sleep has been linked to mental and mood problems such as depression.

In a study conducted in 2014 at the Stanford University School of Medicine, researchers found a connection between lack of sleep and suicide. The study was conducted over a span of ten years. Twenty out of the four-hundred twenty participants who committed suicide reported having troubles with sleeping.

As it is incredibly plain to see with a relatively small amount of research (yet the more research you do, the findings will be the same) that not getting enough sleep can have much worse consequences than many of us had originally thought.

Being tired, feeling less alert and not as quick on the draw, having a shorter fuse and feeling less equipped to adequately deal with everyday life problems, it turns out, are among the most minor of the effects of chronic lack of sleep.

Chapter Three: The Stages of Sleep

"To achieve the impossible dream, try going to sleep" – Joan Kempner

Once a person has fallen asleep, there are five stages of various kinds of sleep to pass through to complete a cycle. Each stage of sleep lasts anywhere from five to fifteen minutes, with a complete cycle lasting anywhere from ninety to one-hundred and ten minutes. These cyclical stages of sleep are broken down between Non-REM Sleep and REM Sleep. REM is an acronym for Rapid Eye Movement, that deepest form of sleep when we are doing the most dreaming. Following are the various stages of sleep and their descriptions:

<u>Stage 1</u>

Stage One sleep is the earliest phase of sleep and can be moved into and out of easily. Did your father use to "doze" in the recliner but snap to as soon as you changed the channel from the football game he'd been watching to the program you had hoped to watch? There's a pretty good chance dad was simply in stage one. This is that form of sleep where one has just "drifted off," and can be easily disturbed by movements or noises. Muscle activity is slow during stage one sleep. Additionally, some people, during stage one asleep, experience occurrences of jerking wide awake, as if from sort of involuntary muscle contraction. Some people have reported that this happens to them simultaneously with a brief sensation that they may be "falling." A person's eyes will still move slowly during this first phase of sleep. Often when a person is awakened from this stage of sleep, they were not even aware that they were asleep at all.

Stage 2

When a person is in stage two sleep, their eye movements stop. Brain waves slow down, with only occasional bursts of more rapid activity. The heart rate slows as the body starts to prepare for a deeper level of sleep. At this time the body temperature begins to drop.

Stage 3

Stage three sleep also referred to as deep sleep is characterized by extremely slow brain waves (called delta waves.) These deep slow waves are occasionally interrupted by smaller faster waves. Stage three sleep is known to be when behaviors called parasomnias occur. Parasomnias are abnormalities experienced by people as they sleep. Included in the parasomnia categories are phenomenon like bedwetting, talking while asleep, sleepwalking and "night terrors" which is a form of panic and similar to what one might experience during a bad nightmare.

Stage 4

This fourth stage of sleep is simply deep sleep. It is characterized by almost non-stop delta waves, virtually non-interrupted by faster brain waves. When one is experiencing stage four sleep and is abruptly awakened, it is normal for the person to feel a sense of confusion or disorientation.

Since stages three and four are considered deep sleep, they are believed to be the most restorative and healing of the sleep stages. In 2008 scientists who study the stages of sleep collectively decided to eliminate stage four sleep, as stages three and four are virtually the same. I've chosen to keep them separated here for comparison of the slight differences.

During stage four, Human growth hormone is produced and contributes to the rebuilding and restoring of stressed muscles. Athletic coaches and experts have long known this. During very difficult workouts the muscles in the body are broken down so they can then be built back up. While this is a very important part of the process of getting stronger, perhaps the more important process is the rebuilding and building back up of stronger muscles in reaction to the stress placed on them. That is why serious athletes or any athlete for that matter must have quality sleep to fully benefit from the vigorous efforts they put into training.

The immune system rebuilds itself during these deep phases as sleep as well, and that is why getting plenty of sleep has always been linked to good health, and when, when a person becomes ill, sleep is highly recommended as an active part of the healing process.

Deep sleep is indeed the most restorative sleep of all the stages.

Because of the depth of sleep obtained in stage three and four, a person who naps during the day will often be less likely to sleep well at night. This is why it's often said that if you're tired during the day to take a twenty-minute "cat-nap." Such a short nap can give you rest and restore you to a point without interrupting or interfering with your sleep cycle later not. This is often easier said than done, rising after just twenty-minutes, as it can feel so nice, and for some people seems relatively easier to drift into a deeper sleep in the afternoon. This comes with the territory of some sleep disorders, such as insomnia, which will be discussed in more depth later.

Depending on the individual, of course, the four stages of sleep as discussed above are estimated to occur from anywhere to four to seven hours per night.

REM

REM (rapid eye movement) is the phase of sleep typically entered in to within about ninety minutes of drifting off to sleep. Many different things occur physiologically within the REM stage of sleep. For one thing, the eyes move rapidly back and forth beneath a person's eyelids...thus the name given to this phase.

Also during this phase, brain activity spikes, blood pressure rises, body temperature cools, and the body enters into what is referred to as a kind of temporary state of paralysis. Since most dreaming takes places during this phase, and certainly the most intense forms of dreams, scientists have set forth the reason for the muscle paralysis as a kind of safety net, should a person awake during a vivid dream and perform rapid, jerky body movements that could ultimately be injurious to the dreamer.

REM sleep is not the only time during sleep when dreaming can occur, but it is when most dreams occur and generally when the most vivid of dreams take place.

It has long been debated as to whether or not everyone dreams. It has become more conclusive with research that all humans do, in fact, dream. How often, how vivid, and whether or not they can remember the dreams after awakening are variables. Another interesting fact is that some people dream in color while others only in black and white.

Chapter Four: What Happens Without Enough Sleep?

"I love sleep. My life has the tendency to fall apart
when I'm awake, you know?"
— Ernest Hemingway

It is a modern myth, although a common one, that it's okay
to exist long-term on very little sleep. In reality, the list of
negative things that can be caused or exacerbated from lack
of sleep is an extremely long one. The list includes side
effects of sleep deprivation from being in a bad mood to
dying prematurely. There are many things that can happen
in between. In this chapter, we'll examine some of the
findings on detrimental effects of not getting enough sleep.

It's safe to say that many Americans can be considered
sleep-deprived, many on an ongoing basis. We are truly a
nation of go-getters and doers. Millions work forty hours
per week at a minimum, some as much as twice that.
People work swing-shifts and graveyard-shifts and still
have families to take care of during the day. Long-haul
truck drivers are expected to cover thousands of miles in
time frames that do not allow for sleep.

The modern lifestyle, or much of it for many people, is not
conducive to getting enough sleep. Most people must get up
in the morning by anywhere from 5:30 to 7:00, depending
on their geographical proximity to work, and what time they
have to be there. The average time spent at work is nine
hours, with one hour considered a "lunch" break that some

may or may not take advantage of. If work starts at eight and ends at five (assuming no overtime) and there's a function that evening at one's child's school, or maybe a going away party to send off a co-worker on their last day at the office. It's clear where I'm going with this. There are hundreds of different job scenarios, but even taking the typical workday, add anything else to it and suddenly there aren't enough hours in the day for all those things to be accomplished with time left over to grab seven or eight hours of sleep before doing it all again.

In this economy, many people are forced to work two jobs simply to survive. Many single parents find themselves in that position. Also, many people work and attend college simultaneously. For college students, the average one at least, in a day filled with work, school, a need to study and a need for sleep, which one do you think is likely to get sacrificed? And, particularly for college students or other people of that age, weekends are not friendly in the catching up on sleep department. Usually quite the opposite. Sleep is the first thing to go out the window in lieu of a good college dorm party!

Reasons for sleep deprivation are endless. Young parents are often up half the night with fussy babies or sick older children. Many children do not like to go to bed and avoid having to sleep. For some parents of small children, bedtime is an unpleasant ordeal every single night. A third-grader, according to research, should ideally be getting twelve hours of sleep per night. In a busy, working parent household, dinner often doesn't even hit the table until eight p.m. Then there are chores like bathing and getting things ready for the next day, clothes to be laid out, and lunches to make. Don't forget to take into account how much children love their television and video games. Many parents allow those things in their children's bedrooms and do not consistently monitor whether or not a child is still watching television or sleeping at eleven p.m. So, if a third grader isn't getting to sleep until eleven, and rising at seven to get ready for school. That's eight hours of sleep, a luxury most of us adults will kill for on an average night, but for a still-growing and developing brain and body, eight hours isn't enough yet and because of these facts thousands and thousands of children's head off to school in the morning deprived of sufficient sleep to set them up for a successful day.

People tend to see sleep as the thing that can be sacrificed when time is pinched. Teens and adults alike. Some people even sacrifice sleep for relaxation time. This is probably a better scenario than being on the run. Rest is not the same as sleep but it can restorative. When I was a single mother, working and going to college, after the work was done for the day, job, homework, chores, daughter put to bed, that was "me" time. That's when the Novel of the Week came out of the drawer on my bedside. I was quite the voracious reader, and I used it as a tool to unwind and prepare for sleep. Yet it's often hard to put an enjoyable book down. If it was already eleven p.m when the book came out of the drawer, it was not uncommon for it to be two the next morning when I, finally exhausted, closed it for the night. Since most mornings I would have to be up and at it by 6:30 a.m. that made for a whopping four and a half hours of sleep. I did this to myself a lot. I was young! It was seemingly without consequence for the most part, and yet was it?

Studies have shown that a lack of adequate time spent sleeping can affect adults in all sorts of negative way. Risks of accidents and injury are increased. It is estimated that six-thousand car accidents are caused each year directly due to people driving while tired. Statistically, one out of twenty-five people falls asleep at the wheel once per month.

It's difficult to pay the proper amount of attention to the road while driving when exhausted. Much like texting and driving, or even drinking and driving, it is flat out dangerous to you and the other drivers and pedestrians out there.

Mood is another thing that can be directly impacted by lack of sleep. For many people, the kind of mood they are in has a huge correlation to how rested they feel. A lack of sleep can easily put someone in a foul mood, shorten their temper and patience, and can make them feel more generally negative about ordinary situations.

Being chronically tired can affect your weight, and lack of sleep has been directly linked to obesity. Sugar is a natural "upper," so it's normal when we're feeling low on energy to reach for junk food. Not just food, but coffee as well. Science now tells us that coffee, in moderate amounts is not necessarily bad for our health. However, for people who drink some of the coffee "concoctions" served at coffee shops, there are incredibly high amounts of sugar in those drinks, and they are certainly not good for our weight or overall health.

While we're talking about caffeine, it is important to remember that while the moderate use of caffeine can give us a physical and mental boost throughout the day, too much of it can trigger a vicious cycle. If you're needing to drink caffeine practically all day to keep yourself going when you decide it's time to sleep the caffeine in your system is going to disagree. Less sleep, tired the next day, more caffeine to survive equals: a vicious cycle.

Lack of sleep can even affect your bottom dollar. Those coffee drinks and office vending machine treats are not cheap, and that money adds up over time.

In certain people, too much sleep deprivation can even lead to drug abuse. According to one study, Adderall is the most abused prescription drug in America. College students abuse this "study" drug, often staying awake for days at a time to make it through finals. Although it is prescribed to treat Attention Deficit Disorder, it is a true amphetamine and has gained popularity even as a street drug.

Immunity to illness is also linked to sleep. By not getting enough sleep, you are compromising your own immune system. This pertains to things as small as the common cold to problems as severe as cancer.

There are other facts to get you thinking about trying to get more sleep. One of them is that lack of sleep affects your judgment, so you may not even realize you aren't getting enough.

Chapter Five: Sleep Disorders

"I'm an insomniac. My mind works the night shift." - Pete Wenz

The topic of sleep disorders is one in which many more thousands of words could be written on what is not known or understood than what is.

Despite all of the studies done through all the years, there's a startling lack of conclusiveness. According to research, there are eighty types of sleep disorders. Yes, you read that number correctly. I will not even attempt to list them all. Instead, the focus of this chapter will be on the most common sleep disorders, affecting the most people.

Approximately seventy million Americans, at any given time, suffer from one or another form of sleep disorder.

Below is a list of seven common sleep disorders:

- Sleep Apnea
- Insomnia
- Restless Legs Syndrome
- Narcolepsy
- Delayed Sleep Phase Disorder
- Rapid Eye Movement Behavior Disorder
- Sleep Walking

Here we'll examine, briefly, what these sleep disorders are and address the most common ways to treat them.

Obstructive Sleep Apnea and regular Sleep Apnea

Sleep Apnea is the second most common sleep disorder and also the most dangerous of all of them to have. Obstructive Sleep Apnea is the most common subtype. Sleep Apnea is a chronic disorder. It affects the body by causing literal pauses in breathing while a person is asleep. The pauses, of course, are extremely brief, but at the same time a person with this condition may stop breathing up to one-hundred times per night, and cause the sufferer to wake often. A common trait of those who deal with this disorder is that they never feel rested, even when they feel like they slept. The problem inherent in the respiratory system shutting down is the brain needs to constantly remain on high-alert over a situation that could potentially deadly. This leaves very little time for someone with Sleep Apnea to reach the truly restful "deep sleep" phase which is the most naturally restorative and responsible for the sense of well-being one feels upon awakening from a good night of sleep.

Obstructive Sleep Apnea (OSA) occurs when the muscles in the throat become blocked ("obstructed") during sleep. Regular Sleep Apnea is caused by a disconnect between the brain and the muscles. The brain fails to send the correct signals to the muscles that control our breathing. Sometimes the two types occur in combination. In those cases, it's called Complex Sleep Apnea Syndrome.

Central Sleep Apnea often occurs from some type of disorder in a person's heart. However, it can also be caused by certain types of medications. Opioids, known to be dangerous in excessive amounts can cause sleep apnea due to their function of slowing down one's respiratory rate. That's why opioids are so dangerous, and the slowing of the breathing caused by them (often when combined with other drugs that suppress the rate of breathing) is generally the cause of death after an overdose.

Obesity is a large contributor to Obstructive Sleep Apnea. As many as half of those who suffer are obese or overweight. Losing weight can contribute to the improvement of and even the elimination of OSA.

Loud snoring, followed by gasping is the biggest sign for how to know if you might be suffering from Sleep Apnea. However, without a partner to inform you, of course, you might not know. The second most recognized symptom is feeling exhausted and dozing off in the day even though you have the subjective feeling that you got a full night's rest.

Sleep Apnea can be diagnosed at home with a portable monitor given to you by your doctor. If you do suffer from this condition, take heart. It is highly treatable. Wearing a CPAP (continuous positive airflow pressure) mask at night is the main treatment, although there are additional options if you find it uncomfortable.

Insomnia

Insomnia is the most common sleep disorder suffered from worldwide. Volumes could be (and have been written) about the nature of this particular beast. Ninety-percent of the population has experienced insomnia at least once or as a temporary condition. Ten percent unlucky members of the population deal with it chronically.

Simply put (although there's nothing simple about it) insomnia is defined as a difficulty falling asleep and/or remaining asleep. It can occur in people of all ages, even children although much less so. It's more common in women than in men and more likely to happen to people as they get older, although many experiences it as a lifelong condition.

Chronic insomnia can exist as a part of another sleep order, or on its own entirely. There are many things that can cause insomnia and many things that can be changed to try to fix it. These things do work in different individuals to different extents, but there are also true people in the world who simply struggle on a continual basis with insomnia despite having tried seemingly everything.

As a normal matter of course, after a doctor has ruled out Sleep Apnea as the cause of insomnia, sleep hygiene will be the next topic of discussion.

Sleep hygiene is made up of the habits we practice around sleep as a whole. If you suffer from insomnia, it is highly recommended that the first thing you do is analyze (and change if necessary) a few basic behaviors. Here are some notes on sleep hygiene:

Your bedroom should only be used as a place to sleep. In other words, the bedroom is not a place you should watch television, use your laptop, play video games or spend time on your phone perusing social media sites, etcetera. The idea is to "train your brain" to recognize that when you get into your bed at night, it's time to sleep.

Make your bedroom and your bed clean, cozy and uncluttered. Consider it your "safe" place. Invest in good sheets and a nice comforter and pillows. Keep decor minimal, using colors you find peaceful and relaxing.

Go to bed at approximately the same time every night, and rise at the same time in the morning. Do not take naps during the day if you can help it.

Do not eat within three hours of bedtime or consume caffeinated beverages after three p.m., even earlier than that for some.

There are many other things that can be done behaviorally to try to help insomnia. Many supplements are out there for you to try. For some, something as simple as a cup of chamomile tea might help. There are also things like Kava Kava and melatonin.

Melatonin is a chemical naturally produced within our bodies in the highest amounts at night when it's time for sleep. Some people simply don't produce enough.

If you suffer from insomnia, do your research. Try listening to sleep hypnosis. It really does work for many people. If you have tried all the behavioral suggestions and the supplements, don't be afraid to talk to your doctor about experimenting with sleep medication. There are many different options.

Melatonin: Melatonin, that sleep hormone that is secreted in our bodies when night falls and its naturally time for us to sleep, is available in a supplement form. Sometimes, for reasons unknown the body simply does not produce enough of this hormone and adding to it with a supplement can be just the thing.

I've had time when melatonin supplements worked for me and other times when they didn't. I ran across an article once that stated that a study had shown that when using Melatonin as a supplement to help with sleep, less is more. Melatonin supplements are sold in capsules or pills, or even sublingual drops in several different dosages. From personal experience, better results were achieved with a two-milligram dose than with five milligrams. You can experiment for yourself, of course.

Purchase a superior quality brand of Melatonin from a reputable seller. I always read the reviews and look at the ratings online to give me an indication of the quality of these types of products prior to purchasing them. Recommendations from friends are great as well.

Kava Kava

This is an herbal remedy made from the roots of a plant called Piper methysticum, found growing on islands in the Pacific Ocean. Natives of these islands have used the plant for medicinal purposes for hundreds of years. It is used to promote calm and relaxation and is also believed to be a mood elevator. Kava might be something to consider if you suspect that anxiety might play a role in your difficulty sleeping.

Again, always buy from a reputable manufacturer and be sure to do your research. Kava Kava is not indicated for use in children under twelve, nor is it considered safe for pregnant or lactating women. It's also not recommended, through some studies, to be used for longer than a three-month period.

Kava Kava can be brewed as tea, taken in capsule form or purchased as a tincture.

Valerian Root
This one is an herb, grown in Europe but also in parts of Northern America. Medicine is made from the root. Valerian is commonly used to treat insomnia.
Additionally, it used as anxiety, so again, if racing thoughts are part of the issue that is keeping you awake, this may be a good one to try.

Research says that doses of anywhere from four-hundred to nine-hundred milligrams of Valerian extract taken up to two hours can be useful in helping you fall asleep faster, and sleep longer.
There are some supplements online that combine all three of the above-mentioned products. That is something you could try as well.

Calcium and Magnesium

Magnesium plays a key role in our ability to sleep, so you want to be sure you're getting enough, whether it's from food sources such as leafy greens, pumpkin seeds, almonds or wheat germ, or taking it as a supplement.

Calcium and magnesium together at night have been proven to have a relaxing effect, and thus could promote sleep.

Lavender Oil

This oil has very calming properties. That's why you will find so many products for babies, lotions and such, that contain lavender. It can be used in many ways. You can add lavender oil to a nice warm bath a little while before bed, or you can put a few drops of essential oil on your pillow.

L-theanine

This amino acid found in green tea leaves may help combat anxiety that interferes with sleep. A 2007 study showed that L-theanine reduced heart rate and immune responses to stress. It's thought to work by boosting the amount of a feel-good hormone your body makes. It also induces brain waves linked to relaxation.

Your Diet

Don't try to go to sleep on either a very full stomach or an empty one. You should eat a healthy dinner at least three hours before bedtime. Should you find yourself getting hungry and it's close to bedtime, it's okay to have a small snack thirty minutes or so before you try to sleep. Keep it light and try to include some healthy carbohydrates and a little bit of protein. An ideal snack along those lines might be a small banana with a tablespoon or two of protein, or a few healthy crackers and a couple of small slices of healthy cheese.

As you can see, there is no shortage of over the counter home remedies for those who are having trouble sleeping. In fact, there are many more than the ones mentioned here for you to try if you care to do your homework and track them down. Also, friends and family are often useful resources. You never know what someone has tried that might work for you.

Remember, as you work your way through the myriad choices of home remedies, if you continue to struggle and nothing seems to be working there are prescription medicines that can help.

While prescription sleeping medications are not a fix, they can serve as a band-aid. Sometimes all that is needed is a little help getting regulated.

Restless Leg Syndrome

Over three million people per year suffer from this strange and terribly uncomfortable condition. As the name suggests, people with RLS feel a constant pretty much irresistible need to continually move their legs, mostly when sitting or lying down.

There are medications for this disorder, but according to modern medicine, there is no cure of yet. If this happens to you and it's extremely bothersome and keeps you awake at night, you will need to see your doctor and be prescribed medication.

This condition has been known to affect children as young as three years old but is generally seen in adults.

Narcolepsy

Narcolepsy is a chronic neurological disorder directly affecting the brain's ability to control sleep-wake cycles. Those who have Narcolepsy generally feel rested after waking, but end up feeling heavily sleepy throughout much of the day. While some people with Narcolepsy seem to sleep okay at night, many experiences interrupted sleep, waking often throughout the night or waking much too early without being able to go back to sleep.

Narcolepsy can take years to be properly diagnosed. That's why it's always good to do as much research as you can if you have a particular area of sleep or daytime drowsiness that you are struggling with. Always go to the doctor armed with as much of your own input as possible. Doctors aren't physics and often being correctly diagnosed is a team effort.

The most common symptom of Narcolepsy is persistent daytime sleepiness, as mentioned above. There are other symptoms that can occur, though they are much more rare.

Three very rare symptoms of Narcolepsy (and reasons for immediate doctor visits) are:

- Sleep Paralysis: A very brief (but terrifying) inability to speak or move which occurs either while falling asleep or waking up.

- Vivid Hallucinations: Again, these primarily occur while falling asleep or waking up. The nature of the hallucinations can be very disturbing.

- Cataplexy: This is a sudden loss of muscle tone (while awake) leading to a temporary loss of control over one's muscle movements. Because of the nature of Cataplexy is sometimes misdiagnosed as a seizure disorder. These attacks range from being mild to being severe enough for a person to collapse.

Delayed Sleep Phase Disorder

This disorder makes it very hard for a person to fall asleep at night. It differs from regular insomnia because once asleep, the sleep is deep and the quality is good. The problem inherent in this condition is that the sleep is so good when its time to wake up school or work it's almost impossible to do so. In these people, their circadian rhythm is off. This disorder is considered part of a family of sleep disorders known as CRSD (Circadian Rhythm Sleep Disorders.) This disorder is often treated with a combination of behavioral modification and medication.

Rapid Eye Movement Behavior Disorder

If you will recall reading earlier about the REM phase of sleep, this is the phase in which we dream most vividly, and also during which we are essentially paralyzed. That paralysis is for our own safety, lest we should "act" on our dreams and cause injury or harm to ourselves or another while sleeping.

In RBD, this natural protective paralysis is absent. Thus this disorder is characterized by the acting out of vivid, often disturbing and sometimes violent dreams.

The most common symptom of Narcolepsy is persistent daytime sleepiness, as mentioned above. There are other symptoms that can occur, though they are much more rare.

Sleep Walking

This condition, which is exactly as the name implies...getting up and walking around while sleeping, occurs more often in children although it does occur in adults. When someone is sleepwalking their eyes are open, so it is a rather eerie phenomenon to witness. Often a sleepwalker will even respond when spoken to, although no always coherently. It is not recommended to wake someone who is walking in their sleep. The best thing you can do is gently get them to go back to bed.

People who walk and/or talk in their sleep typically do not remember it the next morning. If your child is a sleepwalker there are several things you can do to keep him or her safe. Make sure the environment around your child is safe and free from any potentially or harmful objects. Place some type of bell or alarm that will sound to alert you should your child's bedroom door open in the night.

Definitely seek medical advice if the behavior is persistent and troubling.

While by no means inclusive of all sleep disorders, not even close, the above information will help give you a general idea about some of the most common ones. If you are experiencing other difficulties remember, research as much as you can. If the problem seems like something you can work out on your own, give it an earnest try. If you continue to have difficulty don't hesitate to make a doctor's appointment. Good sleep contributes to good health in ways too numerous to list. Sleeping problems should never be ignored.

Chapter Six: Human Circadian Rhythms and Sleep

"We have made clocks that are perfectly in sync with the industrial machinery and the Information Age and perfectly out of sync with nature and our circadian rhythm." – Khang Kijarro Nguyen

Circadian rhythms are physiological, behavioral and mental changes that work on a twenty-four-hour cycle. These rhythms are responsible for releasing the hormones needed at the right time for us to sleep and to wake. Another way to think of a circadian rhythm is to imagine it as your sleep/wake cycle or body clock.

Chronobiology is a word used to describe the process of studying circadian rhythms. With few exceptions, every single organism on the planet follows a circadian clock. The biology of circadian rhythms is incredibly complicated. My hope is to explain them simply enough for the layperson and not put anyone to sleep!

A circadian rhythm pertains to much more than sleep, although light and darkness play a primary role in a circadian cycle. Thus, we are programmed to sleep when it's dark and be awake when it's light. Your personal circadian rhythm dictates what times of the day you will feel most alert, or the most tired.

Our circadian rhythms change to keep up with the lesser

need for sleep we have as we age. Just as you read about earlier, an infant or a teenager will require more sleep than an adult, and older adult requires even less. The natural circadian rhythm changes as we age to reflect our biological needs.

If you could follow your body's own natural instincts about when to sleep and when to wake, you would be more in balance. However, for many reasons already discussed and many more too endless to name, our needs to accomplish certain things do not always jibe with our bodies' natural rhythms. However, if you can incorporate lifestyle changes to better match your body's own rhythms that would be huge. According to studies, following lifestyle practices that healthy circadian rhythms could help you in terms of cognition, alertness, coordination, sleep, of course, heart health and even regularity of your bowel movements.

Have you ever heard the term "Biological Clock?" A Biological Clock is different from a circadian rhythm, in fact, our biological clock is responsible for regulating the timing of our circadian rhythms. A Biological, or Master clock is technically defined as a pair of cell populations found in the hypothalamus, known as the suprachiasmatic nuclei or SCN. These are the actual cells that contain the genes that govern our circadian rhythms.

The brain's circadian clock regulates sleeping and feeding patterns, alertness, core body temperature, brain wave activity, hormone production, regulation of glucose and insulin levels, urine production, cell regeneration, and many other biological activities. The most important hormones affected by the circadian clock, at least insofar as they affect sleep, are melatonin (which is produced in the pineal gland in the brain, and which chemically causes drowsiness and lowers body temperature) and cortisol (produced in the adrenal gland, and used to form glucose or blood sugar and to enable anti-stress and anti-inflammatory functions in the body).

Letting our circadian rhythms dictate our patterns is so important to our overall health it can actually be a factor in an increased lifespan.

Biological clocks that run fast or slow can result in disrupted or abnormal circadian rhythms. Irregular rhythms have been linked to all sorts of different chronic health conditions: sleep disorders, depression, bipolar disorder, seasonal affective disorder, diabetes, and obesity.

The body's "master clock" is in charge of the production of melatonin, the hormone responsible for making us tired. This happens when incoming light is processed through the optic nerves and pass on information from the eyes to the brain. At night, when there is less light, the brain efficiently manufactures melatonin to make you tired and fall asleep. When people lay in bed staring at the light on their smartphones, they aren't doing themselves any favors in terms of promoting natural rhythms. The light from the screen passes through the optic nerves and can throw a wrench into the efficient production of melatonin.

Light, in fact, is a very large component within a circadian rhythm. The deepest instincts within us stem from back to the caveman days. In fact, just as there is a way of eating called the Paleo Diet, with the word Paleo referencing our earliest ancestors, there is an idea set forth about a term referred to as "Paleo Lighting." It's another way to improve our lives by doing what cavemen did. This sounds somewhat counterintuitive since cavemen had it rough, and by anyone's standards we're doing just a bit better, the fact is that very few cavemen (I would be willing to bet) ever suffered from insomnia. Paleo lighting simply has to do with as getting as much bright and natural light during the day as possible to send the signal to your body that it is, indeed, time to be awake and alert and functioning at a high level. Fresh air is wonderful as well, so if you can get outside in the bright light for as little as twenty minutes a day, you are likely going to feel the benefits.

If you happen to live in a cloudy, gloomy locale, there are box lights that can be purchased for the purpose of treating Seasonal Affective Disorder, which is a disorder thought to be linked with light and circadian rhythms. These lights can be used at home or during the day at work. If you choose to go this route, a general guideline is to purchase a light that generates 2,000 lux or more.

Paleo Lighting also suggests you maximize darkness around bedtime and sleep. Remember, caveman did not have lamps, or cell phone screens. One of the worst things you can do when trying to regulate your circadian rhythm is to stare at the bright artificial light of your phone screen for two hours before you try to sleep. It's no small wonder, so many of us have trouble falling asleep.

All kind of things can interrupt circadian rhythms. Often, people who do shift work end up having to take medication to help them remain alert. Since we are programmed to sleep at night, it can be extremely difficult for our bodies to not become "confused" when we try to operate in the opposite way.

Traveling can also interrupt these rhythms, thus the expression "jet lag." Passing into different time zones, your biological clock will be keeping different time from the local time. This can throw you off and make you feel extra tired. Fortunately, our biological clocks are highly adaptable, and they will reset themselves to the appropriate condition.

All of these rhythms vary from person to person based on age, genetic and environmental differences. Our chronotypes, otherwise known as our natural inclinations, are what we need to lead ourselves to the healthiest conditions possible.

The nicest then you can do for yourself is to establish a consistent routine and follow it seven, yes seven days per week. The sacrifice you might see yourself making by giving up "sleeping in" on weekends if that's something you do, will pale in comparison to the benefits you could see if you could get on and stay on a consistent routine.

What that routine will be will be specific to you and the needs of your body and of course your own biological clock. As a matter of course, most humans begin to secrete the "sleep" hormone, melatonin at around 9:00 p.m. and stops it somewhere around 7:30 a.m. During the day, virtually no melatonin is secreted. That's one of the simple reasons why shift workers struggle. People who work a graveyard shift are forced to go against their bodies own nature.

Attempting to do your sleeping during that period when the most melatonin is excreted will set you up for success better than any other thing you can do. Not everyone will have the luxury of being able to retire for the evening by 9:00 p.m., but the closer you can get to the target the better off you will be. It may be difficult at first, but if you can establish a consistent routine, you have a very good chance of improving the quality of your sleep overall. For instance, you will wake less often during the night.

Our eating habits are important in this process as well. Aim to eat the biggest meals the earliest in the day, and studies suggest that it's helpful to keep your eating inside of a 12-hour window. So, for instance, if you eat breakfast at 8:00 a.m., theoretically it should be the biggest meal of the day, followed by a somewhat smaller lunch and light dinner prior to 8:00 p.m. Personally, I would restrict that window a bit more. Eating a meal at 8:00 p.m. and attempting to go to sleep at nine is not the ideal situation. If you can eat earlier, that's always better.

Our circadian rhythms and the way they dictate the release of other hormones can also be a factor in feeling stressed out, and worn out. Cortisol is a hormone secreted by the adrenal glands. As part of a natural circadian rhythm, our cortisol levels are at the highest in the early part of the day when we require extra energy to get moving. The levels continue to rise somewhat throughout the day until finally, they peak then begin to decline and reaches its lowest when it is time to sleep. Excessive amounts of stress can cause a disruption in this process. Cortisol promotes wakefulness, so it's not a hormone we want an elevated level of in our system at night. During a "fight or flight," situation cortisol is released rapidly into the bloodstream. If you experience sudden acute stress like an accident would cause, that feeling of adrenaline rushing through your body can be good, it can help you react.

However, if you have too much stress, your body will begin to release too much cortisol at the wrong times. This not only causes sleep problems but it can cause a condition called Adrenal Fatigue.

If you find you've been under a lot of stress, and that it's affecting your sleep and you're experiencing fatigue during the day, or depression, it would be a good idea to visit a doctor or a Naturopath. There are supplements you can take to help heal your adrenal glands and regulate the production of cortisol. Supplements like Zinc, B6, Magnesium and Vitamin C. A Naturopath can set you on a course of how much of these supplements to take and how often to maximize their healing properties.

If you are experiencing stress or anxiety and it's affecting your sleep, there are other things you can experiment with. Some remedies for different sleep disorders have already been touched on here, but anxiety, or daily life stressors, aren't always factored in as much as they should be when it comes to having problems sleeping. When we worry, our brains will not shut down. Our heart rates stay elevated. These are not conditions conducive to sleep.

If you've never tried meditation, it is a good thing to consider if you have stress in your life. Yoga is great as well. You don't have to go to a class or see a therapist to try some basic meditation though. You can find good instructional videos on YouTube, and you can even download meditation apps on your smartphone. You can always read a book about it as well. Whatever works for you but it has been proven, when even practiced a little bit, to help reduce stress.

A simple meditation exercise I like to do at night is one that focuses on breathing. As a part of my personal sleep hygiene practice, I keep very dim, soothing light in my bedroom. In fact, none of the lights in my bedroom are bright. If I need to during the day, I can open the curtains and let the natural light do its thing. I like candles at night. Sometimes, after a difficult day I will soak in a hot bath with only candlelight about an hour before bedtime. It's not recommended to do this too close to bedtime because part of ideal sleeping conditions pertains to the cooling of our body temperature. I have learned to keep my bedroom very cool. It works best for me, although I realize it's an individual preference.

I have made a hard and fast rule for myself that I do not use my electronic devices when I'm in bed. So, I do my writing and my Facebook perusing and whatever of those sorts of things I need to do prior to going to bed at night. I don't have a television in my bedroom. If I want to watch television (personally I seldom do) I do that in the living room while relaxing on the sofa. The only thing I will do while lying in bed, as part of an evening ritual to relax myself, is read or listen to sleep hypnosis.

There are some really great sleep hypnosis recordings, and while at one time I tended to scoff at such things, I'm now definitely a believer.

Another thing I do, which again, is part of my personal regimen and may or may not be something you find beneficial, is to run a small fan in my bedroom all night. I like the feeling of a little bit of air on me while I sleep, or attempt to, but primarily I do it to create white noise. White noise has always been a factor in creating a comfortable sleep environment for me. Some people use recording of things like rain, or waves lapping the beach. Any of that is fine. Again, sleep hygiene is unique, and it's all about whatever works for any given individual.

I hope more than anything that this book has given you the understanding you were looking for about the science behind sleep, and our circadian rhythms and had placed emphasis for you on how important sleep really is to our overall health.

Life is too wonderful to waste. If I know, there is something I can do to improve the quality of my life I'm going to put the effort in to doing the researching and making my best attempt to apply the principles accordingly. Sleep is truly life-giving. Getting the proper amount of sleep can add years to the time you get to live. Extra years you are allowed the privilege of spending with your children, your grandchildren, your husband or your cats. Whatever your individual case may be. So given that, I will share with you the simple mindfulness meditation I do to help my rhythms and improve the quality of my life. I hope you will give it a try!

This simple exercise will give you an understanding of the concept of mindfulness. Try this first thing in the day, and again at night as you are attempting to fall asleep. Prior to beginning, don't allow yourself to shift any of your focus to all the things you know you need to accomplish across the span of the hours ahead. None of that needs to be of any consequence because it doesn't exist yet. Your day will unfold before you, and you will accomplish your objectives, but you aren't there yet. In this perfect moment, your awareness and focus should begin and end with simply you, your awareness, and your breath.

Start breathing and exhaling slowly, as you normally would in a calm state of mind. Just pay attention to the breathing. Breathe as you normally do.

Notice the way you breathe. Are you breathing in through your nose and out through your mouth? It doesn't matter. There's no right or wrong way to breathe. Just think about your breath as if it were the only thing that matters. Count the seconds it takes you to inhale, then do the same when you exhale. How many seconds total did the cycle take? Six seconds? Ten? You are simply breathing, there's no technique. Let it flow naturally. Allow it to be effortless, like taking in the beauty of a breathtaking sunset.

Your breath is the essence of your existence. Try to hold your attention on it. Should your attention wander, it's perfectly fine. Simply notice that your mind has wandered away from your breathing and bring it back.

Imagine that as you are breathing in you are pulling in to yourself all of the positive energy you will need for your day. As you exhale, picture that breath leaving your body, carrying away any energy or focus you don't require at that exact moment.

Do this for one minute. It's okay to use a timer if you'd like. As you experience the calming nature of this exercise and realize the power it has to bring you sharply back in to the present at any time you choose to use it, you may find that a longer amount of time spent on this practice first thing in the morning is beneficial to you, or break it up and do it several times throughout that day. There are no set rules.

So, if that works for you great, if not that's perfectly okay. There are plenty of things you can do, little rituals you can create for yourself in your personal sleep hygiene routine. I wish you the best of luck for however you choose to approach it!

Conclusion

Congratulations on making it through to the end of *The Science* of Sleep. Let's hope it was informative and able to provide you with all of the tools you need to achieve your goals, whatever they may be.

Sleep in itself, as I have alluded to in this book is somewhat of a mystery by its very nature. After years of extensive research and with over two-hundred sleep clinics in the United States, there are still many questions that have not been answered.

My biggest hope is that by reading this book, you will have come to some realizations, or at least learned some things you hadn't known before.

The take away should definitely be this: Sleep is Imperative! Do not neglect your sleep. If you have children, work with them to help them get adequate amounts of sleep.

It's an ironic situation that people sacrifice sleep so as not to miss out on life, and yet sacrificing too much sleep can actually shorten the duration of a person's life by literally years.

If you do not have a sleep disorder to the degree that you require medical treatment, definitely investigate for yourself the home remedies or supplements I have shared with you. Practice good sleep "hygiene." Turn your bedroom into a shrine to good sleep.

We are all ultimately responsible for our own self-care. By focusing on getting enough sleep, not only are you caring for yourself, you're truly giving yourself an invaluable gift.

Sweet dreams!

Finally, if you found this book useful in any way, a review on Amazon is always appreciated!

Description

In this book, you will discover much about sleep you probably didn't know. This book delves into the most important issues around sleep in easy to read detail.

If you are curious about the nature of sleep, as in how much we actually know about what sleep is, the purpose it serves in our lives and what happens when we don't sleep enough you have ordered the perfect book.

Inside this book, you will find, in addition to other information:

- Guidelines for how much sleep humans need in different stages of their life

- Details about some of the most prevalent sleep disorders, what they are and how they affect people and also the treatments available to them.

- Results of sleep-related research...how sleep affects our health

- Information about the stages we pass through as we sleep

- A description of what is meant by the term "Circadian Rhythm" and how this rhythm affects how you sleep.

- Holistic home remedies you can try for mild or occasional insomnia

Sleep is indeed a fascinating topic to read about. In our modern world, it is so common for people to lead such packed lives. In fact, vast numbers of people pack their lives too full. Something must give, and often times the extra hours that are so badly needed to get through the day are stolen from sleep.

Before there were nine-to-five jobs and even before there were schools to attend, and of course prior to the invention of electricity, people slept entirely based on the rhythms of their bodies. And, because there was no such thing as "processed foods' people ate much better as well.

Since the early 1800's humans have come light years in terms of progress. Scientists have been discovered and been able to accomplish and achieve so much in terms of our health and overall well-being. However, in part because of that progress we seem to have gone backward where sleep is concerned.